Safe at Home
'Home Safety Edition'

Protecting you and yours in and from your home™

by Randy DeVaul

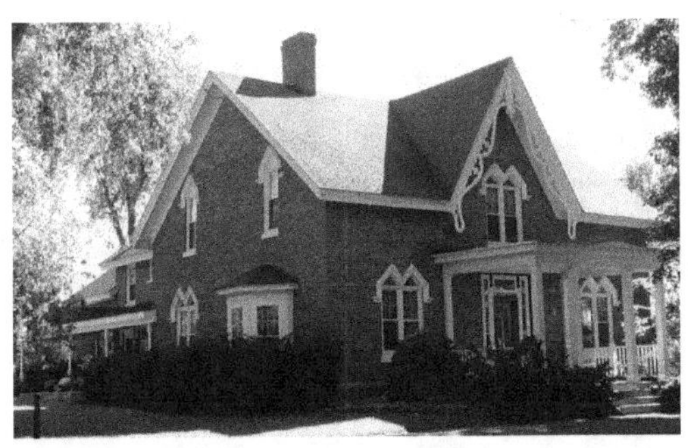

Safe at Home
'Home Safety Edition'

Protecting you and yours in and from your home™

by Randy DeVaul

Published 2014

Published by Brickhouse Press, a Division of Brickhouse of NY, Inc,
7573 East Route 20, Westfield, NY 14787, USA.

Manufactured in the United States of America.

About the Author

I have been a safety professional and an emergency response provider and instructor for more than 30 years. I have both witnessed and responded to needless, preventable injuries and fatalities directly related to family members taking risks that should not have been taken. Sometimes, these family members knew the risks and believed they could beat the odds. Other times, the risks or hazards were 'hidden,' meaning they were not seen or perceived as dangerous. Regardless, the end result was the same.

The information in this booklet can help you, the reader, and your family to identify common and hidden risks and hazards so you avoid any injury or incident from occurring. Using a common sense approach and real-world examples, my goal is to help you prevent a needless and preventable event from occurring to "protect you and yours in and from your home™."

Randy DeVaul's Workplace Safety books and e-books:

Performance Safety: A Practical Approach
Performance Safety: Above and Beyond
Performance Safety: Lessons for Life
Performance Safety: Lessons for Life eBook

Home Safety e-book titles available:

Home Safety: Boating Safety
Home Safety: Around the Home
Home Safety: Home Emergencies
Home Safety: Healthy Living (food, nutrition)
Home Safety: Holidays Year Round
Home Safety: In the Home
Home Safety: Room to Room
Home Safety: RV and Camping
Home Safety: Summer Fun
Home Safety: Winter Wiles

Preface

This book is a compilation of safety articles from the 'Safe At Home' column. The purpose of this book is to help illuminate the common and the hidden hazards associated with home emergencies.

These articles relate to topics that expose real life-threatening hazards. The information is provided in an easy-to-read, informal tone with practical, real-world experiences and tips for preventing a fatal mistake from happening.

INTRODUCTION

Thanks for purchasing this Home Safety Edition. This contains information on Home Emergencies, Home Safety Room to Room, and Holiday Safety topics. The additional included report provides information on discounts often available from homeowner and renter insurance companies when a household has the items listed in the report. If you don't know of the discounts and have these items or you want to ensure more of your family's safety by getting these items for your home, contact your insurance provider and ask if a discount applies once these items are within your home.

If you find the information in this book helpful, please feel free to email me and let me know how it helped. With your permission, your shared story could be in the next book! Email me at safetypro@roadrunner.com.

Thanks, again, and have a great day!

Randy DeVaul

BOOK 1: HOME EMERGENCIES

TABLE OF CONTENTS

BOOK 1: HOME EMERGENCIES

Fire!

It is time to change the clocks and check those batteries in your smoke detectors. If you fail to change your clocks, you might not show up at the right time. If you fail to change your smoke detector batteries, you might not show up at all!

Fires are the third leading cause of accidental death, so protecting you and your family from such a tragedy is necessary. As you set your clocks and check your batteries, take just a few extra minutes and check for these fire prevention conditions in your home.

I hope you have smoke detectors so there are batteries to check. They are not expensive and strategically placing two or three throughout the house make good sense. There should be at least one on every floor of the house and, at the very least, one in the hall near the bedrooms and one near your kitchen. The kitchen detector is important, especially if someone turns meal preparation time into burnt sacrificial offerings.

While in the kitchen, check (or purchase) a small fire extinguisher rated for grease fires. It is easy to become distracted while cooking between the phone, the kids, the pets, the neighbors, or simply reading the recipe for the next ingredient. If the extinguisher is more than a couple years old, you may want to replace it.

Have you checked the lint trap in your dryer lately? The lint trap filter should be pulled and cleaned after every couple of uses of the dryer to prevent dangerous build-up of lint. It only takes a few seconds to do it.

Make sure your fireplace and chimney are clean from soot and other partially-burned material. If you haven't checked your flue in a while, you may also end up with the fresh-grilled aroma of wildlife that moved in during the off-season. Don't mix wood logs with commercial chemical logs since popping of hot embers and potential explosion of material can occur. Don't burn wrapping paper or color-coated catalog pages. Not only can they cause a rapid flare-up of flame, but they also give off dangerous toxic fumes and smoke.

Kerosene and other types of heaters should be away from other things that burn, such as wall paper, drapes and curtains, upholstered furniture, and electrical cords. And of course, don't use gasoline in any of your heaters or fireplace!

If you smoke, quit! Yes, I know that is easier said than done. Burning cigars and cigarettes have burned many homes to the ground from ashes dumped in trash containers or falling on upholstered furniture. You see, dumped or fallen ashes do not immediately cool. The heat can work on other materials when smoldering. You go to bed or leave the room, and two hours later you have a fully-engulfed fire!

These suggestions only take seconds to check and doing so can save you and your family's life. Don't take your safety for granted. Take the time to be safe at home!

First Aid Starter Kit

Are you ready for an injury at home? Be prepared for home emergencies with a properly stocked first aid kit. You can purchase one commercially or design and stock your own. Not all items in commercial kits are necessary. Get formal first aid training so you know how and when to use your kit's components. These items make for a good basic starter kit:

Durable storage box/bag
¾ inch bandage strips (Band-Aids or similar)
2" x 2" sterile gauze pads (for use with wound cleanser)
4" x 4" sterile gauze pads
2" wide roll gauze (non-sterile)
Hypo-allergenic adhesive/bandage tape
Small bandage scissors
Small tube of antiseptic/antibiotic ointment
6 triangular bandages (for slings or securing gauze pads)
Wound cleanser solution (hydrogen peroxide or similar)
1 pair tweezers
Small individually packaged alcohol wipes for hand cleaning
2 pair disposable gloves
2 junior size cold packs
2 zip-lock sandwich bags
Penlight-size flashlight (disposable or with batteries)
Bottle of saline solution or eye wash
Pre-packaged emergency blanket

If small children are in the house: a small bottle of activated charcoal and syrup of ipecac (only use under the direct instructions from the Poison Control Center)

Don't stock burn ointment! If a burn occurs, use cool water or use ice that is not placed directly on the skin to alleviate the pain of the burn. Cover the burn area with a dry sterile dressing and, if blistered or charred, seek medical attention. Do not use rubbing alcohol to cool a burn since it may cause too much heat to be removed from the body as it evaporates.

Don't stock splints. If you are not trained to use them you will only cause further pain and discomfort to your loved one. Don't stock pain relievers, antacids, etc. This is not your medicine cabinet!

Some items have expiration dates so check the kit regularly to ensure contents are current and that the flashlight still works.

In addition to these listed materials, you may need items such as medicine dispensers, spare hypodermic needles, and other personal items. Do not store medications requiring refrigeration.

Keep the first aid kit accessible, yet away from young children. If professional medical help is needed, call 9-1-1 and keep the patient comfortable while waiting for help to arrive. If you suspect something is broken, do not move it. Simply allow your patient to sit or lie comfortably and treat for shock.

Treatment for shock includes: loosening tight or binding clothing; covering the patient to protect from excessive heat or cold; if it won't aggravate the injury, prop your patient's legs up about 8" off the ground. Do not give food or drink as this may cause vomiting (your patient, perhaps, followed by you).

I hope you will never need these items. Having them available in one place, however, prepares you for a quicker response in an emergency and helps you be safe at home.

Grab-n-Go Bag: On the Run

When a disaster occurs, you do not have the luxury of time to gather critical items to take with you. Nor is it the time to decide what to do with your pets. All of that should be determined before the event, in a disaster or emergency plan.

Whether tornado, fire, flooding or other quickly occurring event, you need to protect your family and respond rapidly. With guidance from the Federal Emergency Management Agency and the American Red Cross, here is a checklist for your "Grab-n-Go" kit.

Ahead of time:
learn local evacuation routes and locations of public shelters
learn of any special assistance available for people with special needs (elderly, disabled, medical treatments, etc.)
determine fate or location of pets (animals generally not allowed in public safety or housing shelters)
learn first aid and/or CPR
create a personal/family emergency plan if required to evacuate, including a meeting or assembly location for family members if you get separated
program your cell phone's speed dial with 'ICE' (In Case of Emergency contact phone number)
prepare a "Grab-n-Go" kit

"**Grab-n-Go**" Kit suggested contents:

duffle bag, backpack, suitcase or other suitable container
a contents list with any expiration dates noted
supply of water (one gallon per person per day) – rotate/replace every 6 months
supply of non-perishable packaged or canned food and a non-electric can opener
change of clothing (including underwear and extra socks)
water-repellent jacket or rain gear
toiletry kit of travel-size deodorant, toothpaste, toothbrush, shampoo, soap, sanitary napkins, if needed
blanket(s) or sleeping bag(s)
small flashlight(s), portable radio, extra batteries for both

extra pair of glasses (take glasses over contact lenses to avoid cleaners, etc.)
credit cards and cash (if electricity is out, credit card accounts and ATMs cannot be accessed)
an extra set of car keys
phone numbers of relatives or friends in state and in another state (for widespread disasters)
a list of family physicians and extra or copies of health insurance card(s)
a photo identification
a copy of each Social Security card, birth certificate, vehicle title
special items for infants (diapers, bottle(s), formula, a toy), elderly, or disabled
a list with serial number(s) for medical devices, such as pacemakers

If you have time as you leave:

shut off electricity, gas, water at main switches/valves
put on or take a pair of sturdy shoes (not your bunny slippers)
contact a friend or relative to tell them when and where you are going

In your vehicle, have:

booster cables
pack of emergency flares
extra blanket(s)
small shovel
5-lb. fire extinguisher
First aid kit
Maps or road atlas
Small packs of bottled water and high-energy foods (granola bars, peanut butter, raisins, etc)
Cell phone battery charger (AC and DC capabilities)

Advance planning can keep you and yours safe at or away from home.

ICE Your Cell Phone

A growing trend in cell phone use is the ability to program an emergency contact phone number in the event of an unplanned injury or other emergency. Many of us with cell phones have numbers programmed into speed dial along with the 9-1-1 number. But what happens if you are unable to use your cell phone because of an injury or serious illness?

Your speed dial numbers may include friends, distant relatives, and professional contacts all mixed in with family numbers. An emergency service provider attempting to contact your designated emergency contact will not know which of those numbers, if any, should be called if you are incapacitated. Searching through a cell phone memory of numbers takes valuable time and without a way to identify the emergency contact person from the list of stored numbers, the wrong person or no person may get contacted to advise of your situation and location.

An idea initiated in Great Britain is spreading quickly across the Atlantic and becoming an accepted means of cell phone use during an emergency. To identify your emergency contact on your cell phone, simply program the letters I-C-E in front of the name of the person to call.

I-C-E stands for 'In Case of Emergency' and it quickly tells emergency responders or hospital providers who to contact if you are unable to tell them. Though not officially adopted as the 'preferred means' of providing emergency contact information, it is becoming very popular in the United States amongst emergency responders as well as other systems across the globe.

There are databases and other systems that have been developed over the years, especially after 9/11 here in the United States. Some of those systems, however, require a fee to utilize with on-going subscription rates. The I-C-E system is free of charge to every cell phone user and is getting more and more exposure for putting it in use.

There are a couple safety or security concerns: one is that you are identifying your emergency contact and phone number. In the event of your phone being lost or stolen, that number would be in someone else's hands for potential prank calls. One way around that is to get the location name and phone number of where your loved one is supposed to be, then immediately call operator assistance to verify the number and the location.

Another problem is if the person's number is not up-to-date or you change your emergency contact without changing it on your phone. I can't imagine it taking too long for someone to recognize that the wrong name or number is programmed, but it is something to consider.

When you finish this article and before you do anything else, go program I-C-E into your phone to identify your emergency contact person. Then, should something happen to you that prevents your ability to use your phone, you know your contact can be notified in a timely manner and you can feel more secure and safe at home.

Prepare for the Worst!

This is not a "gloom and doom" article. Rather, it offers tips for expecting, planning for, and getting through emergencies while protecting yourself and your family.

First, create a simple plan. Professionals use an all-hazards approach to emergency planning and response. You will need to know how to respond to three types of emergencies – medical (injury or illness), weather (taking shelter), and evacuation (getting out of your house).

If a medical emergency occurs, call 9-1-1. Don't ever hang up; stay on the phone with the dispatcher. Most likely, the dispatcher will remain on the line with you to help you through the event while waiting for help. Show younger children how to dial the phone and explain to them in a calm way how and when they should call the emergency number. Use the cell phone as a last resort as most dispatchers can determine your address by the caller ID with your phone number.

Whether day or night, turn on the outside light to your house and advise the dispatcher that it is on. This helps the emergency crews locate your home quicker when looking for the address. If you have pets, place them outside in the back yard or in a room where you can close them in behind a door. This will ease the tension of the responders as well as protect your pets.

Dangerous weather requires making a decision. Can we stay in a safe place in the house (basement, crawl space, inner room away from windows) or do we need to go (or have time to go) to a community shelter?

Create a space in your garage, basement, or closet to keep a home emergency box or kit. Call your local American Red Cross chapter for help with kit contents. But be sure to include, batteries, flashlights, candles, matches, a battery-operated radio, a couple blankets, some canned goods that don't require cooking, a can opener, and bottled water, to name just a few items.

Create a checklist so you don't forget things like baby formula and diapers, medications, a spare pair of glasses, relative's phone numbers, perhaps a change of clothing.

If you need to evacuate your home due to fire or other emergency, identify a place outside of the house where everyone should gather. Establish a fire escape route and review with your loved ones (seniors and children) what they should do. Run a practice drill and make it fun for your kids so they don't panic. That way they'll know what to do and where to go in a real situation.

Don't forget to plan for your pets. They usually can't go to a shelter with you so pre-planning for them rather than leaving them to fend for themselves is important.

There is never a bad time to plan for an emergency. Children, senior adults, and everyone in between must know what to do before an emergency occurs. Plan now to help you cope with the incident and keep your family safe.

Your Home Emergency Checklist

Are You Ready?

Emergency Planning and Checklists from the Federal Emergency Management Agency

Prepare your family by creating a family disaster plan. You can begin this process by gathering family members and reviewing the information you obtained in Section 1.1 (hazards, warning systems, evacuation routes and community and other plans). Discuss with them what you would do if family members are not home when a warning is issued. Additionally, your family plan should address the following:
Escape routes.
Family communications.
Utility shut-off and safety.
Insurance and vital records.
Special needs.
Caring for animals.
Safety Skills
Escape Routes
Draw a floor plan of your home. Use a blank sheet of paper for each floor. Mark two escape routes from each room. Make sure children understand the drawings. Post a copy of the drawings at eye level in each child's room.

Where to Meet
Establish a place to meet in the event of an emergency, such as a fire. Record locations below:

	Where to meet...
Near the home	For example, the next door neighbor's telephone pole
Outside the immediate area	For example, the neighborhood grocery store parking lot

Family Communications

Your family may not be together when disaster strikes, so plan how you will contact one another. Think about how you will communicate in different situations.

Complete a contact card for each family member. Have family members keep these cards handy in a wallet, purse, backpack, etc.

You may want to send one to school with each child to keep on file. Pick a friend or relative who lives out-of-state for household members to notify they are safe.

Create a **contact card**. A copy should be in your family disaster supplies kit.

Utility Shut-off and Safety

In the event of a disaster, you may be instructed to shut off the utility service at your home.

Below is some general guidance for shutting off utility service:

Modify the information provided to reflect your shut off requirements as directed by your utility company(ies).

Natural Gas

Natural gas leaks and explosions are responsible for a significant number of fires following disasters. It is vital that all household members know how to shut off natural gas.

Because there are different gas shut-off procedures for different gas meter configurations, it is important to contact your local gas company for guidance on preparation and response regarding gas appliances and gas service to your home.

When you learn the proper shut-off procedure for your meter, share the information with everyone in your household. Be sure not to actually turn off the gas when practicing the proper gas shut-off procedure.

If you smell gas or hear a blowing or hissing noise, open a window and get everyone out quickly. Turn off the gas, using the outside main valve if you can, and call the gas company from a neighbor's home.

CAUTION - If you turn off the gas for any reason, a qualified professional must turn it back on. NEVER attempt to turn the gas back on yourself

Water

Water quickly becomes a precious resource following many disasters. It is vital that all household members learn how to shut off the water at the main house valve.

Cracked lines may pollute the water supply to your house. It is wise to shut off your water until you hear from authorities that it is safe for drinking.

The effects of gravity may drain the water in your hot water heater and toilet tanks unless you trap it in your house by shutting off the main house valve (not the street valve in the cement box at the curb—this valve is extremely difficult to turn and requires a special tool).

Preparing to Shut Off Water

Locate the shut-off valve for the water line that enters your house. It may look like the sample pictured here.

Make sure this valve can be completely shut off. Your valve may be rusted open, or it may only partially close. Replace it if necessary.

Label this valve with a tag for easy identification, and make sure all household members know where it is located.

Electricity

Electrical sparks have the potential of igniting natural gas if it is leaking. It is wise to teach all responsible household members where and how to shut off the electricity.

Preparing to Shut Off Electricity - Locate your electricity circuit box.

Teach all responsible household members how to shut off the electricity to the entire house.

FOR YOUR SAFETY: Always shut off all the individual circuits before shutting off the main circuit breaker.

Insurance and Vital Records

Obtain property, health, and life insurance if you do not have them. Review existing policies for the amount and extent of coverage to ensure that what you have in place is what is required for you and your family for all possible hazards.

Flood Insurance

If you live in a flood-prone area, consider purchasing flood insurance to reduce your risk of flood loss. Buying flood insurance to cover the value of a building and its contents will not only provide greater peace of mind, but will speed the recovery if a flood occurs. You can call 1 (888) FLOOD29 to learn more about flood insurance.

Inventory Home Possessions

Make a record of your personal property, for insurance purposes. Take photos or a video of the interior and exterior of your home. Include personal belongings in your inventory.

You may also want to download the free Household and Personal Property Inventory Book from the University of Illinois to help you record your possessions.

Important Documents

Store important documents such as insurance policies, deeds, property records, and other important papers in a safe place, such as a safety deposit box away from your home. Make copies of important documents for your disaster supplies kit. (Information about the disaster supplies kit is covered later.)

Money

Consider saving money in an emergency savings account that could be used in any crisis. It is advisable to keep a small amount of cash or traveler's checks at home in a safe place where you can quickly access them in case of evacuation.

Special Needs

If you or someone close to you has a disability or a special need, you may have to take additional steps to protect yourself and your family in an emergency.

Disability/Special Need	Additional Steps
Hearing impaired	May need to make special arrangements to receive warnings.
Mobility impaired	May need special assistance to get to a shelter.
Single working parent	May need help to plan for disasters and emergencies.
Non-English speaking persons	May need assistance planning for and responding to emergencies. Community and cultural groups may be able to help keep people informed.
People without vehicles	May need to make arrangements for transportation.
People with special dietary needs	Should take special precautions to have an adequate emergency food supply.

Planning for Special Needs
If you have special needs: Find out about special assistance that may be available in your community. Register with the office of emergency services or the local fire department for assistance so needed help can be provided.

Create a network of neighbors, relatives, friends, and coworkers to aid you in an emergency. Discuss your needs and make sure everyone knows how to operate necessary equipment.

Discuss your needs with your employer.
If you are mobility impaired and live or work in a high-rise building, have an escape chair.

If you live in an apartment building, ask the management to mark accessible exits clearly and to make arrangements to help you leave the building.

Keep specialized items ready, including extra wheelchair batteries, oxygen, catheters, medication, food for service animals, and any other items you might need.

Be sure to make provisions for medications that require refrigeration.

Keep a list of the type and model numbers of the medical devices you require.

Caring for Animals
Animals also are affected by disasters. Use the guidelines below to prepare a plan for caring for pets and large animals.

Guidelines for Pets
Plan for pet disaster needs by:

Identifying shelter.
Gathering pet supplies.
Ensuring your pet has proper ID and up-to-date veterinarian records.
Providing a pet carrier and leash.
Take the following steps to prepare to shelter your pet:
Call your local emergency management office, animal shelter, or animal control office to get advice and information.
Keep veterinary records to prove vaccinations are current.

Find out which local hotels and motels allow pets and where pet boarding facilities are located. Be sure to research some outside your local area in case local facilities close.

Know that, with the exception of service animals, pets are not typically permitted in emergency shelters as they may affect the health and safety of other occupants.

Guidelines for Large Animals
If you have large animals such as horses, cattle, sheep, goats, or pigs on your property, be sure to prepare before a disaster.

Use the following guidelines:
Ensure all animals have some form of identification.

Evacuate animals whenever possible. Map out primary and secondary routes in advance.

Make available vehicles and trailers needed for transporting and supporting each type of animal.

Make available experienced handlers and drivers. (Note: It is best to allow animals a chance to become accustomed to vehicular travel so they are less frightened and easier to move.)

Ensure destinations have food, water, veterinary care, and handling equipment.

If evacuation is not possible, animal owners must decide whether to move large animals to shelter or turn them outside.

Also see FEMA's Information for Pet Owners for help on protecting and caring for your pet during an emergency.

Safety Skills
It is important that family members know how to administer first aid and CPR and how to use a fire extinguisher.

Learn First Aid and CPR
Take a first aid and CPR class. Local American Red Cross chapters can provide information about this type of training. Official certification by the American Red Cross provides, under the "good Samaritan" law, protection for those giving first aid.

Learn How to Use a Fire Extinguisher
Be sure everyone knows how to use your fire extinguisher(s) and where it is kept. You should have, at a minimum, an ABC type.

For additional assistance, see FEMA's Disaster Supplies Checklist.

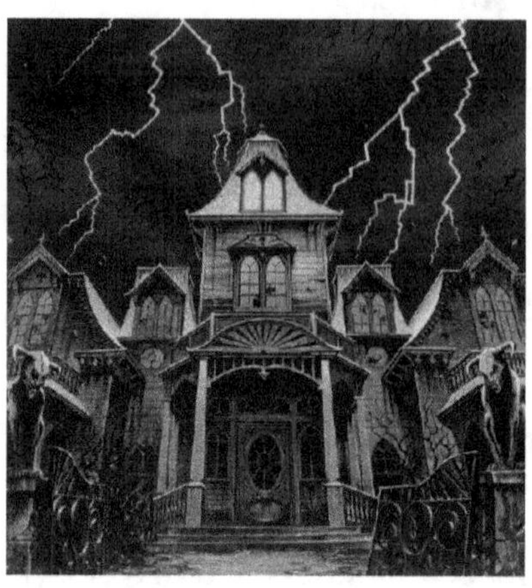

BOOK 2: HOME SAFETY ROOM TO ROOM

TABLE OF CONTENTS

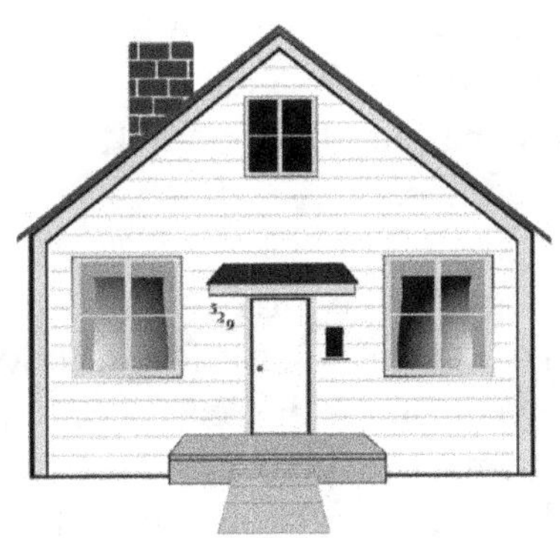

House Tour – Surviving Your Home

These series of articles will take us on a whole 'house tour.' The purpose of this tour is to identify common, yet oftentimes hidden, hazards that we encounter every day inside our 'castle' walls and yet, continue to stay alive by somehow avoiding mayhem and death.

The tour begins with a general hazard overview around the house. As you enter your front door, what do you see? Is the entry way clear of obstacles and toys or do you have to walk into the house with both eyes peeled to the floor to avoid skates, balls, the dog, or other trip and fall hazards? Check to see if there is enough lighting at the door and easily accessible inside the door as you enter. You may want a motion-type sensor switch so the room or entry light comes on as you enter. If it is also light-sensitive, it will only come on when it is dark so you can just leave it on.

Head for the kitchen and see if you can quickly locate the kitchen fire extinguisher and that you can actually get to it without removing half your closet of clothes hanging from it. Look to ensure the gauge is 'in the green,' fully charged and ready to go. Look up and make sure your smoke alarm is in place and working. Uh-oh – you don't have a fire extinguisher or smoke alarm in the kitchen? Get one for under $20 and call your insurance carrier to say that you have one. It could give you a discount on your homeowner's insurance.

Do you have leftovers on the counter or some in the refrigerator you can no longer identify? Toss them! Don't forget to look under the sink to see how easily your three year old or dog can access all of your toxic goodies; then either relocate them elsewhere or find a way to secure your floor-level cabinet door to keep kids and pets out of there.

The living area should be free of multiple-plug extension cords, cables, candles, or 'stuff' around your electric baseboard heat. Do you walk through the house still wearing your shoes? If so, what might you be carrying on to your carpet fibers from work or out on the street? Kids should be positioned at least three feet back from the television and check the volume to ensure you are not causing deafness in the family.

Moving on to the most popular part of the house – the bathroom – check to see if you have a secure bath mat near the tub rather than just slippery

wet flooring when you step out of the tub or shower. You should have GFCI electrical receptacles so you won't get electrocuted plugging in the hair blower or shaver and don't forget to push the 'test' button from time to time to make sure it actually works.

From here we'll take a closer look at each room. See you next time.

House Safety Tour: The Kitchen

The kitchen is one of the most dangerous rooms in the house. Aside from the potential of killing the family through burnt offerings, there are numerous other hazards that must be recognized in order to eliminate the fatal or injurious consequences.

The most obvious preventable hazard in the kitchen deals with food preparation, storage, and leftovers. Do not cross-contaminate uncooked meats with other foods (great way to spread the unhealthy bacteria). Cook foods to proper temperatures to ensure unhealthy bacteria are 'toast.' Do not leave cooked or refrigerated foods out for longer than two hours (again, the unhealthy bacteria – see a pattern here?). Refrigerate leftovers quickly and be sure to reheat them to proper temperatures before eating them again.

Moving on, have a fire extinguisher in the kitchen with a smoke detector. This is not to make fun of the cook's skill but to ensure if something catches fire – grease, oven-ables, dish towels next to toasters, etc – the detector will get your attention so you can use the fire extinguisher and save having to watch everything you own burn to the ground. That is an experience I am familiar with – it is exciting; it is not fun.

The floor can create slip or fall hazards from wet dishes, liquid spills, or simply leaving a floor-level cabinet door or drawer open and then attempting to walk past it with the casserole dish that just came out of the oven. In addition to the flowery speech that may loudly blurt out (did I say that out loud?), you may be lying in hot food with shards of 'dish' penetrating body parts.

Knives and other sharps, such as pizza cutters, create obvious hazards. If you have children or pets, keep these items out of their pathways. Be careful if doing dishes or removing these items from the dishwasher to reduce the risk of puncture wounds.

Scalds and burns are high on the list for toddlers and small children, though such injuries are not exclusively theirs. Pan handles and other utensils should be positioned so they cannot be grabbed and flung off the burner on the stove. Of course, you don't want to position them to where you have to cross over another hot burner or have the handles 'pre-

heating' prior to picking them up. Pets are also on the scald list as they are usually under foot or close by when the pan or pot gets dropped.

Finally, consider what you are wearing with what you are doing. Loose or dangling sleeves, jewelry, or hair may make your fashion statement, but watching them melt while you are still attached to them is a painful experience. Ladies, engagement rings, particularly the stone settings, are reactive over time to cleaners, detergents, and basic knocking around. Your diamond may be forever but your setting is not. Show some care or you could ingest your diamond with that next mouthful.

Do a quick walkthrough right now and fix what you find so everyone stays safe at home!

House Safety Tour – the Bathroom

If not the most popular room in the house, the bathroom is certainly one of the most visited of all the rooms. For its basic size, it also has the greatest number of hazards per square foot than any other room, except for, perhaps, your storage shed.

Studies show that 70% of home accidents occur in the bathroom. The combination of water and smooth surfaces makes taking a bath or shower particularly dangerous. And you thought your kids simply enjoyed their own body odor over wanting to take a bath. Who knew it was a self-preservation response? Over 100 persons die of bathtub-related burn injuries every year and one person dies every day from using a bathtub/shower in the United States. Bathroom deaths are the second leading cause of accidental death and disability after automobile accidents.

So, what do we do to stay alive when visiting the most used room in the house? Regardless of your age, here are some pointers to ensure you and your family's safety.

First, on a somewhat lighter note yet all too real of identified hazards, consider these real-world events. One of the most common hazards to young boys' genitalia is the toilet seat falling while attempting to go. Smaller children drown by toddling head-first into the toilet bowl. People have dislocated hips from sitting down on the toilet rim without the seat in place. Skin has been pinched and blood drawn from sitting on split plastic seats. Also imagine using the toilet as a stepping stool to reach above your head and having your feet slip out from under you. Ouch!

Grab bars for tubs, showers, and even the commode help prevent slips and falls. Ensure that the flooring remains clean and dry. If using a bath mat to soak up water, make sure that it has grippers on the bottom so it doesn't become a 'slip and slide.'

Before installing non-slip strips to the bottom of your tub or shower, carefully select the right material so they are durable. Some cleaning materials may not be compatible and cause the strips to peel, flake, or otherwise not stick. This creates a real problem if pieces try going down the drain and clog. Many of the newer tubs and showers don't need the added strips.

Medicine cabinets and under-the-sink vanities are marvelous storage facilities for all sorts of toxic, cutting, and otherwise dangerous products. Do not place these items where pets and children can eat or play with them.

Scalding can be a problem if your water heater is set too high. Thermostats are generally easy to adjust. You want the water in your sink and tub to be under 120 F. A nice red ring develops on submerged skin at 110 F.

Electrical hazards are deadly. Newer bathrooms are required to have ground fault circuit interrupter receptacles to the circuit breaks if moisture becomes a factor with your plug-ins. Test the circuit by pushing the 'test' button to know that it still works properly.

House Safety Tour – the Family Room

No matter what you call this room – the den, living room, family room – this is the room where at some point in time everyone in the family will meet and/or entertain friends, family, and themselves. This is often the 'catch-all' room where relaxation is the goal, playtime is the objective, and clean-up is not always on the agenda.

This room usually has bookcases, television or media carts, computer game stands, and various pieces of furniture that include floor and table lamps, end and coffee tables, and extension cords and outlet strips routed throughout the floor along the walls and doorways. These items if not illuminated well or kept from being hidden by clutter offer wonderful opportunities for slips, trips, and falls.

Kids playing and running around can slip and fall into a table corner or trip on a cord that yanks the plug out of an outlet or crashes the lamp to the floor. If using area rugs rather than wall-to-wall carpeting, be sure they are 'gripped' to the floor and not designed for magic carpet rides across the room.

This room is famous for attracting clutter. Toys, game pieces, homework that the dog took the blame for eating all find their way easily accumulating on the floor and the furniture. All of this stuff can create numerous hazards by concealing heaters, cords, and floor space. For those of us who are aging and our eyes are not working the way they used to, well-illuminated rooms are essential to reduce the risk of running into, over, or through something.

Fire hazards develop when combustible materials hide or cover periodically used heaters, such as baseboard or supplemental units. Always be sure to have a smoke detector in the family room and check the batteries a couple times a year – say, when the time changes in the spring and fall – to ensure it is working.

Bookcases and other heavy furniture that is up against the walls should be secured with furniture straps and brackets to keep them upright. Kids and pets love to climb and they can be seriously injured when the top-heavy wall unit falls on them after successfully climbing half-way up.

Monitor the noise levels of televisions, music, computer games, and the like. It doesn't take long for decibel levels to exceed safe limits and staying in an enclosed or re-verbing (echoing) room with everything blaring is a great way to reduce your hearing ability. High noise levels can also create issues with your pets as they desperately attempt to get someplace quieter just to be able to relax.

Between carpeting, pets, and décor plus various holiday decorations and knick-knacks, dust and other compiled materials can become real allergens. It doesn't take long for kids to start breathing funny or develop perpetual runny noses when they are indoors so besides basic dusting, consider an air purifier or something similar to keep on in the room.
The family room is a social gathering spot. Keep it safe and healthy for everyone!

House Safety Tour – the Bedroom

If we are getting enough sleep in the first place, the bedroom is where we spend a third of our lives. For those of us who do projects, homework, and other activities beyond 'sleep mode,' our bedrooms can easily become a major-use room. It just makes sense that it should be a safe haven to ensure a good night's sleep without worry of something going wrong.

First, don't smoke in bed. It takes less than three minutes for a fire to become life-ending. Smoking in bed can be much more dangerous than simply affecting your health.

Housekeeping comes up often but the fact that more than 70% of all injuries are a direct result of poor housekeeping causes me to remind you regularly. Clutter in the bedroom (have you seen the kids' room?) with clothes, shoes, books, and other 'extraneous' floor-level items can create a trip and fall hazard – particularly if needing to get out of the room quickly! If you have baseboard electric heat, built-up dust, clothes, papers, and other combustibles create a real-world fire hazard. Install and regularly check batteries in smoke detectors right outside the room in the hall.

Furniture, such as bookcases and shelving units, dressers, and other free-standing items should be sturdy and not easy to tip over. Do not store heavy items on top shelves – keep them low to the ground to prevent tipping as well as ensuring the heavy stuff isn't so high that you can't get it down without a back and neck injury.

Always have a well-lit closet and room. You want to see where there might be stacked stored boxes that could fall or where trip hazards may be in the room. Also, check closet rods to ensure they are secure and not to high to reach. Consider padding sharp edges of furniture whether in the kids' rooms or in yours if there is a risk of losing balance or falling into them.

Night lights are always a good idea, regardless of the age of the person in the room. You never know when there will be a 'midnight run' (no, I don't mean food in the kitchen) that requires getting to the bedroom door safely.

You have to decide whether you want locks on the bedroom doors – particularly for the kids' rooms. If you do have locks, be sure to have a spare 'master' key that will get you in the room if something happens, whether fire, medical emergency, or other situations.

I need to at least mention that if you have young children, be sure to cover electrical outlets and always locate any supplemental heaters carefully so children do not get burned by contacting them. Of course, additional items such as clock radios, audio equipment, charging cords for electronics, and other plug-ins should be kept clear of the head of the bed to avoid getting wrapped in them and certainly avoid overloading the outlet with too many items plugged into it.

Enjoy your sanctuary and stay safe!

House Safety Tour – Basement/Attic/Storage Sheds

As we look at the storage areas around the house, a number of safety tips apply to each location.

First, these areas should be well-ventilated. If you live in an older home (mine is 170 years old), that may not be a problem. My attic or basement will never be 'air-tight.' For newer homes, keep some airflow just to keep heat, radon, moisture and mold risks, and vapors from stored items at safe and healthy levels.

Housekeeping is critical. Keeping these areas neat and 'navigable' reduce risks of fire, rodent and other wildlife infestations, and trip and fall hazards. Also, be sure to have good illumination so you can safely maneuver.

Depending on the season, heat exhaustion or hypothermia are risks so don't plan an all-day search or clean out during the dead of winter or the height of summer. Finally, make sure you have safe access with sturdy and non-cluttered stairs, handrails, and a light switch located where you start, not where you end up.

The Basement

Do not store gasoline or other flammable contents (mineral spirits, paint thinners, etc) in the basement. Any vapors generated can easily get to the gas pilot light on the furnace or water heater or spark at your electrical panel or fuse box.

As mentioned previously, check radon levels. You do not want to be breathing radon air.

Place a fire extinguisher in the basement – just like the one in your kitchen. Remember, the extinguisher does not make you a professional fire fighter to save your house; it is there to assist you in getting out of the house. Spring for an extra ten bucks and include a smoke detector, as well, placed strategically in the ceiling area.

Moving storage items up and down stairs (including the attic) means you need your stairs to be clear of clutter and your storage items not exceeding your maximum lift abilities. It's a great idea to store things in boxes but remember you still have to be capable of moving them at some point in time. Also remember that as you age, your lifting capabilities decrease so you may have to split a load in a large box to two smaller boxes just to ensure you can safely move them.

The Attic

Keep heavier boxed storage items in the basement. Usually the attic stairs are more narrow, less sturdy, and only wide enough to fit your body through the ceiling hole. Not a good place to try maneuvering awkward boxes.

If you are adding insulation or hooking up an exhaust vent, stay on the rafters, not the floor, or you could end up in your bedroom after falling through.

The Storage Shed

Mowers, plastic gas cans, fertilizers, insecticides, aerosols, no windows and closed door – got a match? Finally, never use your shed as a storm cellar.

Use common sense when storing things, buy only what you need, and don't bulk up on materials you can't use. Keep you, your family, your pets, and your neighborhood safe!

Home Fall Prevention Checklist for Older Adults
Provided by the US Centers for Disease Control

FALLS AT HOME

Each year, thousands of older Americans fall at home. Many of them are seriously injured, and some are disabled. In 2002, more than 12,800 people over age 65 died and 1.6 million were treated in emergency departments because of falls.

Falls are often due to hazards that are easy to overlook but easy to fix. This checklist will help you find and fix those hazards in your home.

The checklist asks about hazards found in each room of your home. For each hazard, the checklist tells you how to fix the problem. At the end of the checklist, you'll find other tips for preventing falls.

FLOORS: Look at the floor in each room.

Q: When you walk through a room, do you have to walk around furniture?
Ask someone to move the furniture so your path is clear.

Q: Do you have throw rugs on the floor?
Remove the rugs or use double-sided tape or a non-slip backing so the rugs won't slip.

Q: Are there papers, books, towels, shoes, magazines, boxes, blankets, or other objects on the floor?
Pick up things that are on the floor. Always keep objects off the floor.

Q: Do you have to walk over or around wires or cords (like lamp, telephone, or extension cords)?
Coil or tape cords and wires next to the wall so you can't trip over them. If needed, have an electrician put in another outlet.

STAIRS AND STEPS: Look at the stairs you use both inside and outside your home.

Q: Are there papers, shoes, books, or other objects on the stairs?
Pick up things on the stairs. Always keep objects off stairs.

Q: Are some steps broken or uneven?
Fix loose or uneven steps.

Q: Are you missing a light over the stairway?
Have an electrician put in an overhead light at the top and bottom of the stairs.

Q: Do you have only one light switch for your stairs (only at the top or at the bottom of the stairs)?
Have an electrician put in a light switch at the top and bottom of the stairs. You can get light switches that glow.

Q: Has the stairway light bulb burned out?
Have a friend or family member change the light bulb.

Q: Is the carpet on the steps loose or torn? Make sure the carpet is firmly attached to every step, or remove the carpet and attach non-slip rubber treads to the stairs.

Q: Are the handrails loose or broken? Is there a handrail on only one side of the stairs?
Fix loose handrails or put in new ones. Make sure handrails are on both sides of the stairs and are as long as the stairs.

KITCHEN: Look at your kitchen and eating area.

Q: Are the things you use often on high shelves?
Move items in your cabinets. Keep things you use often on the lower shelves (about waist level).

Q: Is your step stool unsteady?
If you must use a step stool, get one with a bar to hold on to. Never use a chair as a step stool.

BATHROOMS: Look at all your bathrooms.

Q: Is the tub or shower floor slippery?
Put a non–slip rubber mat or self–stick strips on the floor of the tub or shower.

Q: Do you need some support when you get in and out of the tub or up from the toilet?
Have a carpenter put grab bars inside the tub and next to the toilet.

BEDROOMS: Look at all your bedrooms.

Q: Is the light near the bed hard to reach?
Place a lamp close to the bed where it's easy to reach.

Q: Is the path from your bed to the bathroom dark?
Put in a night–light so you can see where you're walking. Some night–lights go on by themselves after dark.

Other Things You Can Do to Prevent Falls

Exercise regularly. Exercise makes you stronger and improves your balance and coordination.

Have your doctor or pharmacist look at all the medicines you take, even over-the-counter medicines. Some medicines can make you sleepy or dizzy.

Have your vision checked at least once a year by an eye doctor. Poor vision can increase your risk of falling.

Get up slowly after you sit or lie down.

Wear shoes both inside and outside the house. Avoid going barefoot or wearing slippers.

Improve the lighting in your home. Put in brighter light bulbs. Florescent bulbs are bright and cost less to use.

It's safest to have uniform lighting in a room. Add lighting to dark areas. Hang lightweight curtains or shades to reduce glare.

Paint a contrasting color on the top edge of all steps so you can see the stairs better. For example, use a light color paint on dark wood.

Other Safety Tips

Keep emergency numbers in large print near each phone.

Put a phone near the floor in case you fall and can't get up.

Think about wearing an alarm device that will bring help in case you fall and can't get up.

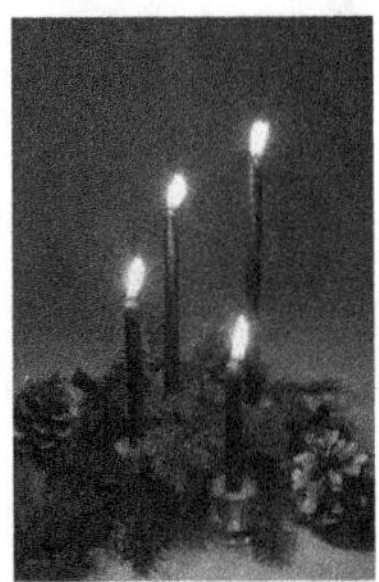

BOOK 3: HOME FOR THE HOLIDAYS

A Date With Danger: Valentine's Day

Celebrating with Fireworks: July 4

Enjoying the Holidays: You and Your Pets

Food Feast or Food Fight: Holiday Cooking

Getting Into the Holiday Spirits - Alcohol

Happy Halloween: At Home and On the Street

Home for the Holidays

And

Your Home Holiday Safety Checklist

TABLE OF CONTENTS

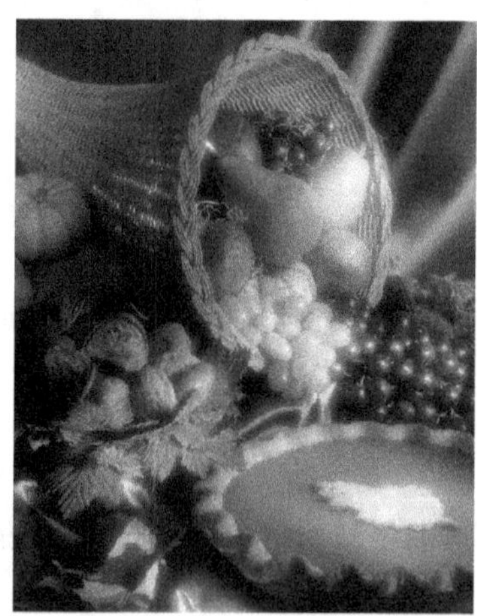

Date With Danger on Valentine's Day

Valentine's Day is the *one* day in the year that let's you show, share and shower love on loved ones with romantic gifts and dinners. It's probably good that there is a special day to remind us guys to recognize our significant other, though the new set of platinum booster cables may not be the gift she had in mind.

You might try cooking something special to show how much you care. The National Restaurant Association reports that about one third of couples actually go out for dinner on Valentine's while the rest work toward preparing a gift of love at home. Of course, this is after the flowers and favorite chocolates have arrived so there is an anticipation of romance for that perfect someone. Put your favorite music on low, light the table candles, and you are ready to serve your loved one a special meal. This is assuming that you can prepare something special or, at least, follow the microwave instructions on the box.

If you are preparing something new for the special occasion, ensure your main course is cooked properly and that it hasn't passed its "sell by" or "use by" date (guys, now is not the time to get that 'great deal' from the 'expires today' sale). How long that meat has been in the refrigerator as well as sitting on the store shelf does make a difference. Otherwise, you and your date may become a statistic from a date with danger from a tiny microorganism called Listeria monocytogenes (Lm), which grows on food even when refrigerated.

And what about dessert? Crème brûlé, chocolate mousse, tiramisu, salmonella – what? Yep, those rich decadent egg-based desserts if not prepared properly can give you and your loved one a real exciting time later that evening.

Do you have pets? I am sure you know how deadly chocolate can be to your animals, as well as certain flowers and plants. Loading up the chocolates and flowers (guys, check for allergies or your evening will end abruptly from airway and nasal issues, something that does not lend to romance) can provide a curious pet with a deadly combination. Veterinarians advise that as little as four ounces of chocolate can kill a ten pound dog or cat. Sharing left-overs with your pet is also dangerous. High sodium or salt in foods can create serious health problems.

Some pets love to eat ribbon and may be very afraid of balloons so take this into consideration before giving these to your significant other or keeping them 'unguarded' around the house. A pet ingesting ribbon can experience life-threatening blockages in airway or in the digestion system. Don't use the pet as an excuse to not give a gift but do take that into consideration.

So, plan ahead. Practice your menu before actually serving it. Use fresh ingredients. Or if you are kitchen-challenged, be part of the one third across America and go out. If you choose to stay home, stay safe at home.

Celebrating with Fireworks

Fireworks are a fun way to celebrate our nation's birthday. We are fascinated by the colors and sounds and often want to participate in creative ways for using them. Too often we forget that we are exposing ourselves, our kids, and our pets to dangerous, even life-threatening, hazards.

One of the most popular items that adults give to children to hold and wave is a sparkler. Since it doesn't explode like other fireworks, we have the false belief that a sparkler is safe for a youngster to use. But no one under five years of age should be given a sparkler and there must always be adult supervision. Bear in mind, sparklers can burn as hot as 1,200 degrees F. Dropping it or throwing it can cause severe burns to bodies and property. Also, once the sparkler stops, place it head down into sand because it is still very hot. People have placed them in water only to find that the water gets too hot and causes burns, as well.

The fireworks most commonly purchased and used at home besides sparklers include whirlers and fountains. Always maintain a safety zone of no less than 6 yards (18 feet). Wear long-sleeved shirts, pants (not shorts) and shoes to prevent burns from spatter, dropping, and shooting of debris. Never go barefoot around fireworks!

The U.S. Consumer Product Safety Commission offers these additional safety tips:

*Do not allow any running or horseplay.
*Light fireworks outdoors in a clear area away from houses, dry leaves or grass and flammable materials.
*Keep water nearby for emergencies and for pouring on fireworks that don't go off.
*Do not relight or handle malfunctioning fireworks. Douse and soak them with water and throw them away.

*Be sure other people are out of range before lighting fireworks.

*Never ignite fireworks in a container, especially a glass or metal container.
*Keep unused fireworks away from firing areas.
*Store fireworks in a dry, cool place. Check instructions for special storage directions.
*Observe local laws.
*Never have any portion of your body directly over a firework while lighting.
*Don't experiment with homemade fireworks.

Remember your pets. Don’t take your animals to fireworks displays. The sudden booms and other unusual noises can cause pets to tremble, shake, howl, refuse food, and even attack simply out of fear and trying to get away from it all. They can also suffer from heart-related problems that can be life-threatening to them.

If using fireworks around the home, do NOT use them close to any animals. Getting too close to exploding fireworks can cause the animals to become victims of burns and eye damage, severe injury, or death. And certainly do not ever throw fireworks at people as a joke.

Have a fun and safe holiday. Keep the pranks and practical jokes for other times and be respectful to others. That way we can all enjoy the fun and beauty of fireworks while ensuring that we and our loved ones (including pets) are safe at home.

Enjoying the Holidays: You and Your Pets

The weather outside might be frightful, but you don't want the inside of your home to be. During the holiday season, we get festive and, sometimes, down-right crazy with lights, decorations, candles, fires, and the like which pushes the safety margin off the scale. For those of us with pets (or maybe young children), we create hazards that can endanger their lives and not even know we have done so.

If you have a dog like mine (or perhaps a 2-year-old) – one that eats and drinks anything first only to wonder later if it was worth it – watch what plants are in your home. Dogs and cats seem to enjoy holly, mistletoe, poinsettias, and lilies but to their detriment. And you get to clean up the deposited contents in various shapes and smells.

Those "gotta have one" snow globes often contain antifreeze so if you drop and break one, clean up the liquid immediately since antifreeze tastes sweet and deadly.

Not so much dogs, but cats love to eat and play with tinsel. Keep the loose tinsel on higher branches and off the floor. A cat that ingests tinsel can cause blockage in the intestines, creating pain and perhaps death while you pay the vet bill.

Ever hear of putting aspirin in your tree stand water to keep the tree healthier longer? Aspirin-laced water can be fatal to your pet. And if you choose to not use aspirin, still don't let your animal drink the water in the tree stand. It can often contain fertilizers as well as pine needles (puncture holes in intestines) and stagnant water breeds millions of interesting little bacteria. You also don't want pets eating (or leaking on) your tree, wrapped gifts, and extension cords, so placing some type of netting or screening around the tree will eliminate a multitude of hazards.

The increased activity and visitors during the holiday season can over-stress your pet. Often times what is a normal routine throughout the rest of the year changes during the holidays and pets (and young children) do not like change. Don't take the behavioral differences out on them (pets or kids) if you are the one causing the problem. Try to maintain regular feeding and exercise schedules and give them (both) a little extra attention so they know they are loved.

Although it may be tempting, don't give in to feeding your pet table scraps during the holidays (or any other time). We are already going to gain an additional 5-20 pounds from over-eating. That is not what you want to achieve with your pet!

A special word from pet groups everywhere, do not give a pet as a gift to someone else. Everyone is under stress during this time of year, including the pet and the recipient. Instead, give pet supplies or gift cards and let the new owner find a more appropriate time to select and care for a new pet. Everyone wins.

From our house to yours, have a wonderful holiday season!

Food Feast or Food Fight: Holiday Cooking

It's time for holiday cooking and all of its trimmings! Are you ready for all of that food? Aside from the fact that Americans between November and January add on the pounds to go with the blessings, there is one way to keep those pounds off. No, not exercise or diet. Not smaller portions. Not choosing to eat out rather than home (that's what buffets are for, right?). No, one method of weight control that should NOT be part of your thinking. It's called foodborne illness – from those little creatures that love to help you see what you already ate!

There are a number of ways to get a foodborne illness and a handful of ways to protect yourself and your family. There are safe ways to purchase, store, prepare, and serve your food as well as safely taking care of the evening graze on the left-overs so you don't encounter the gastro-intestinal disorders, such as the unpleasantness of blowing lunch in either or both directions.

First, when purchasing your materials, always place your meat and poultry items in the shopping cart last and separate them from each other while in the cart and in the bags when going home. Refrigerate these meats as soon as you get home and don't take a side trip on the way. If you thrift-shop for your canned vegetables, be sure to purchase cans that are not dented, cracked or bulging.

Wrap or bag your meat or place it on a plate before placing it in the refrigerator so it doesn't leak raw juices onto other foods. Also make sure the refrigerator temperature stays below 40 degrees F to prevent growth of foodborne bacteria.

According to Michigan State University findings, bacteria are the source of 67% of all food poisonings in the US. These bacteria thrive in food when between 40-140 degrees F for longer than two hours. So preparing it, storing it, and eating left-overs by keeping the food in the proper temperature range is critical! And the most common food handling mistake is cooling food too slowly to place back in the refrigerator.

You may be more susceptible to foodborne illness than others. Children and infants produce less stomach acid than adults, making them more prone for bacteria attack. Pregnant women place the fetus at risk because of an under-developed immune system. Older adults can be more at risk due to poor circulation, reduced nutrition, or from low protein in their diets.

So, don't thaw your meats at room temperature. Don't stuff your turkey the night before. That body cavity insulates the stuffing and produces millions of tiny bacteria. Cook your meats at temperatures above 325 degrees F. Don't let your prepared food set out for day-long munchies. Use good personal hygiene habits. Coughing, sneezing, and body-part-picking does not enhance the flavor.

Enjoy the holidays and all that food. New Year resolutions come after the holidays for a reason. Prepare and eat the food properly so you can be safe at home!

Getting into the Holiday Spirits

With the additional stress, partying, gift giving, feelings of loneliness, and depression increasing during the holiday season, alcohol use increases, as well. The season also generates more air and road travel, making alcohol and traveling ar dangerous mix.

If traveling by plane, for example, drinking alcohol can create problems from discomfort to life-threatening conditions to changes in behavior. It also creates problems for the other passengers and flight crew.

Cabin crews from 206 commercial airlines ranked over-consumption of alcohol at the top of their list of factors that trigger air rage attacks on planes. And, with new security measures slowing down the boarding process, alcohol enhances frustrations from delays, stress, smoking bans, and other factors. For the infrequent air traveler, the stress of just getting on the plane encourages alcohol consumption.

The Aerospace Medical Association states that numerous conditions created within the cabin of an airplane are complicated when alcohol is used. A pressurized cabin, for example, provides an atmosphere equal to being atop a small mountain at between 5,000-8,000 feet. That reduces oxygen levels in the body. Add alcohol and the body's metabolism slows, which slows the breathing rate and heart rate, reducing the oxygen levels further.

Alcohol dehydrates the cells within the body. On long flights, drinking alcohol with the reduced humidity level in the cabin (generally less than 20% humidity) can cause skin and eye irritation, particularly for contact lens wearers. So, increase water intake before and during the flight. Also select water and juices over alcohol or caffeine, such as coffee, tea, and soft drinks.

Exposure to a colder climate with high levels of alcohol in the body can increase the likelihood of hypothermia – a generalized cooling of the body that can become dangerous. To reduce this risk, reduce the alcohol intake while ensuring proper clothing is available to wear once you arrive at your destination. A short-sleeve shirt is no match to standing outside in below freezing temperatures while waiting for the rental car or for public transportation.

Leaving a cold climate for hot can be dangerous when alcohol is involved. The sudden change in temperatures won't allow the body to adapt to the change quickly enough, leading to increased sweating and loss of body fluids. Since alcohol is both a dehydrator and body depressant, a person's ability to adjust to a sudden temperature change can cause problems with the heart, blood pressure, response and reaction time, and slow the decision-making process.

Parties are great for family and friends to celebrate the season and the new year. But don't drink and drive. Alcohol affects work faster when on an empty stomach. Eating something when drinking helps absorb the alcohol and reduce its affects on the body. That alone can help reduce the chance of driving while intoxicated as well as doing something stupid or embarrassing while at the party.
So, this year, have a great holiday season by acting responsibly as we continue to hope for peace on earth and goodwill toward all men!

Halloween At Home and on the Street

Celebrating Halloween with costumes, decorations, and trick-or-treating can be a lot of fun for the entire family! There is no doubt that you will see and maybe do things during Halloween that (fortunately) you will not see or do any other time of the year. To ensure it remains fun for everyone, here are some suggestions to keep the celebration safe and healthy.

First, pre-plan for both your house and your kids. Costumes that are bright and reflective will reduce the tire marks from drivers not seeing 'halloweeners.' Use non-toxic, hypoallergenic makeup in place of full-faced masks to prevent vision and breathing problems. Wigs and costumes should also be flame-retardant. Too many children and adults end up in burn units from pranks and ill-suited costumes.

Outdoor decorations can be really cool, but remember you will have children running across your yard. If you plan to be visited by extra-terrestials, goblins, monsters, royalty and superheroes, remember these children cannot actually fly. Unless, of course, they are flying over your yard stuff from not seeing them. Keep your decorations lit or in non-pedestrian areas (such as front lawns and culverts) to reduce potential lawsuits and prevent injuries. Other items you may not think of include flower pots, garden hoses, low tree limbs or roots, and other house and yard items.

Find accessories for costumes that are flexible and soft. Knives, sticks, swords, and guns – even play ones – can pose life-threatening hazards if your child falls on them or gets him killed in some neighborhoods or business areas if the weapon looks real.

For the main event, have a route or location already established. Many of the malls now offer a safe environment along with costume contests for children, as do other organizations. Make sure you have the right batteries for flashlights. Feed your children a good meal prior to going out to reduce the sugar-meal-syndrome when returning with all of their goodies.

Act responsibly with your pets. Try not to put them outside or in a high visibility area. It not only scares the daylights out of the 'weeners, but can make your pet more aggressive as it believes it is under attack by strange beings. Keeping your pet indoors will also reduce the risk of the pet being attacked or injured by someone.

And finally, the basic list: warn your children about entering people's homes or vehicles; do not let your kids use bicycles, rollerblades, or skateboards; don't let younger children go alone and, if possible, go in 'herds' or groups. That works well for the kids and the homeowners; don't let your children eat anything that is not properly wrapped; only go to homes that have the outside or porch light on.

This is obviously not an all-inclusive list. You can search the internet for "Halloween safety" for more suggestions. Halloween can be fun. Keeping it safe for adults, children, and pets will provide a positive experience for everyone!

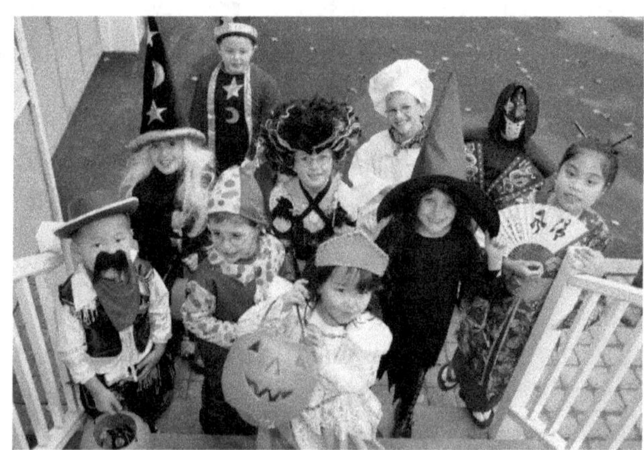

Home for the Holidays

There really is no place like home for the holidays. Especially if you have children. While our children are still at home, our rule is, "If others in the family want to see us, they'll visit us." Of course, it may be harder to get rid of them once they show up. You'll have to weigh the benefits to the challenges on that one.

Anyway, how you prepare your home for the holidays can create memorable family times. Make sure it is not from calling the poison control center or the fire department. So keep the following safety tips in mind.

If you plan to have a real Christmas tree, pick out a healthy one right from the start. A fresh live tree shouldn't lose needles when tapped on the ground. Once in place, give it plenty of water so the needles don't dry up and "flame out." A six-foot tree will use up to a gallon of water every two days! And if you want the tree up way early for the holidays, consider an artificial tree and an aerosol can of "pine tree scent."

According to the National Fire Protection Association, almost half of all fires involving Christmas trees were caused by electrical problems – short circuits, circuit overloads, etc.. So, use miniature lights and do not connect more than three strands of lights together. Many of the artificial trees today have a maximum lights note with the tree so they don't become over-lit. Check the light cords each year. If the cord is frayed or the outside insulation is cracked or peeled, throw the lights away and make a trip to your local "dollar" store. Do not load up an extension cord or wall outlet with more extension plugs. If you need more plug space, use a power strip with a built-in circuit breaker. And always turn off the lights when you leave the room or get ready for bed.

Children and pets can get the shock of their lives, as well. Remember the cat in National Lampoon's Holiday Vacation? It's a scream in the movies; it's a real scream in real life. Placement of lights, glass ornaments, and other decorations in the home must consider the age of the children and temperament of any pets.

Outside decorations can be beautiful. I love those "tacky lights tours" that show-off people's imagination. If you compete this year, here are some pointers.

Make sure your neighbors are up for it. Nothing quite like an abrupt change in your holiday plans from a friendly neighborhood "shotgun party." It may be your right, but you gotta live with your neighbors all year 'round. Use lights and cords designed for use outdoors. And if you are hanging lights from the house, use the right ladder the right way.

Decorating your house for the holidays can be fun. Be sure to stay safe at home for the holidays and not spend it in a shelter or with extended family from fire or other disasters.

Your Home Holiday Safety Checklist

Provided by 'Safe at Home' and
US Fire Administration / Federal Emergency Management Agency

Each year fires occurring during the holiday season claim the lives of over 400 people, injure 1,650 more, and cause over $990 million in damage. There are simple life-saving steps you can take to ensure a safe and happy holiday and reduce your chances of becoming a holiday fire casualty.

Preventing Christmas Tree Fires

Christmas Tree Fire Hazards - Movie segments demonstrating how fast a live Christmas tree can become fully engulfed in flames. Special fire safety precautions need to be taken when keeping a live tree in the house. A burning tree can rapidly fill a room with fire and deadly gases.

Selecting a Tree for the Holiday

Needles on fresh trees should be green and hard to pull back from the branches, and the needle should not break if the tree has been freshly cut. The trunk should be sticky to the touch. Old trees can be identified by bouncing the tree trunk on the ground. If many needles fall off, the tree has been cut too long, has probably dried out, and is a fire hazard.

Caring for Your Tree

Do not place your tree close to a heat source, including a fireplace or heat vent. The heat will dry out the tree, causing it to be more easily ignited by heat, flame or sparks. Be careful not to drop or flick cigarette ashes near a tree. Do not put your live tree up too early or leave it up for longer than two weeks. Keep the tree stand filled with water at all times.

Disposing of Your Tree

Never put tree branches or needles in a fireplace or woodburning stove. When the tree becomes dry, discard it promptly. The best way to dispose of your tree is by taking it to a recycling center or having it hauled away by a community pick-up service.

Holiday Lights

Maintain Your Holiday Lights

Inspect holiday lights each year for frayed wires, bare spots, gaps in the insulation, broken or cracked sockets, and excessive kinking or wear before putting them up. Use only lighting listed by an approved testing laboratory.

Do Not Overload Electrical Outlets

Do not link more than three light strands, unless the directions indicate it is safe. Connect strings of lights to an extension cord before plugging the cord into the outlet. Make sure to periodically check the wires - they should not be warm to the touch.

Do Not Leave Holiday Lights on Unattended

Holiday Decorations

Use Only Nonflammable Decorations

All decorations should be nonflammable or flame-retardant and placed away from heat vents.

Never Put Wrapping Paper in a Fireplace

It can result in a very large fire, throwing off dangerous sparks and embers and may result in a chimney fire.

Artificial Christmas Trees

If you are using a metallic or artificial tree, make sure it is flame retardant.

Candle Care

Avoid Using Lit Candles

If you do use them, make sure they are in stable holders and place them where they cannot be easily knocked down. Never leave the house with candles burning.

Never Put Lit Candles on a Tree

Do not go near a Christmas tree with an open flame - candles, lighters or matches.

Finally, as in every season, have working smoke alarms installed on every level of your home, test them monthly and keep them clean and equipped with fresh batteries at all times. Know when and how to call for help. And remember to practice your home escape plan.

PERSONAL AND MONEY-SAVING REPORT

Safety and Savings: Save Money with Home Safety

Here is a way that you can almost immediately benefit in savings by following some simple, yet life-saving practices. Many insurance companies offer discounts on home premiums with certain safety equipment working in your home. This can be 10-15% off your total premium, generally at an annual savings greater than your Safe At Home™ annual membership!

First, have working smoke detectors strategically placed throughout your home. You don't need one for every room. Consider one for the family room and the hallway leading to the bedrooms. If you have more than one floor, you may want to place one at the top of each stairway, as well.

Install a carbon monoxide detector. It is generally more expensive than a smoke detector but there are combination units available for purchase that are often less expensive than purchasing one of each. Consider a carbon monoxide detector for rooms where you have a fireplace, supplemental heaters such as kerosene, propane, or natural gas, or near ductwork from a gas or oil furnace.

A kitchen fire extinguisher is another item that insurance companies will ask about for the safety discount. Since grease fires are common and dangerous, having an extinguisher readily available in the kitchen provides an extra measure of safety.

Dead-bolt locks increase your security so having these on your entry doors will be favorable for you. Another protective device is a security alarm system for fire or intruder detection. Having one or getting one installed may provide an additional 5% discount with many companies.

In Florida, insurers want to see a windstorm protective system installed on the house. This may include window shutters and other items to protect your home from wind damage, such as an impact-resistant roof. Other states may have requirements, such as a roof made of non-combustible material (something that won't likely burn if a fire is present). Before installing expensive items, such as the security system or windstorm protective system, contact your insurer for recommendations or for which ones will earn you the discount. If you already have these items, tell your insurer.

In summary, most insurers will give some form of a premium discount for basic items that you already have or should have, anyway. These are:

- working smoke detectors
- a kitchen fire extinguisher
- dead-bolted exterior/entry doors
- a carbon monoxide detector for homes with a fireplace or supplemental fuel heaters.

You won't get these discounts automatically – you have to ask for them. So don't be shy – call your insurer and ask about the safety discount. Not sure where to purchase these items? As a convenience, check out SAHI's 'Safety Products' page or visit your local home improvement or discount stores.

Epilog

Thank you, again, for reading. My hope is you gleaned some family-protecting pointers and tips that help you keep you and yours safe in and around your home for years to come.

As I stated at the beginning of the book, if you have a story to share of how something in this book alerted you to a problem that you were able to correct or you learned something you didn't know before that helped you or your family avoid a hazard that was present in your home, please share your story with me. Drop me an email at safetypro@roadrunner.com.

I would be honored if you felt this information was important enough to pass along to others, whether you give this book to someone else or you want to hang on to it and tell others where they can get their own copy.

Have a safe day!

www.ingramcontent.com/pod-product-compliance
Lightning Source LLC
Chambersburg PA
CBHW070614290526
45790CB00002B/910

* 9 7 8 1 5 0 3 2 2 2 3 4 2 *